FITNESS FOR THE MIND AND BODY

FITNESS FOR THE MIND AND BODY

A Holistic Approach to a Better You

CLARA WINTERSHADE

QuillQuest Publishers

CONTENTS

CHAPTER 1

Section 1: Introduction

Of course, among the five factors of human makeup, the body is born and dies as long as Jivatma is alive inside the body. No two bodies are similar in size, color, weight, texture, etc. Thus, the body is phenomenal and the enjoyment is said to be Manomentric. Here, the mind is important. The body without the mind would be lifeless. This is the main reason why the body is alienated by people when they die.

In the same way, if anyone misunderstands the ancient systems and believes they do not indicate anything concerned with the body, it may be dangerous to healthy living with the intent practice of Yoga, Therapeutic and Indian Head Massage, and other alternative systems in countries like the USA and the UK. The beauty of the human personality is derived from the culture of the heart, the unique gift to mankind. At the same time, the human makeup possesses five factors, namely, body, soul, atma, gnanendriyar, and karmendriyarm, which deserve respect from mankind. This is true and does not raise any dispute or controversy among a variety of cultures and life.

Integration is not a new concept. It has always been in existence. Its full form today is called holistic health. No language or practice explicitly explained the concept in a simple and easy manner. It now receives care and application everywhere in the present era. The body is conjoined with the soul and atma, and there is no way to separate it. In case it is separated, the result will be marana or ultimate death. Thus, holism is a significant part of the ancient Indian systems, both spiritually and alternatively.

CHAPTER 2

Section 2: Benefits of a Holistic Approach

There are different ways to define mental health. According to the medical definition, mental health is a manifestation of the individual's emotional well-being. This may be because the individual has worked with a level where they can live normally regardless of any stressful situation or environment. However, the unity of physical and psychological health is possible. Thus, recommendations for the method of achieving and maintaining good mental health are very different because living with a mental disorder can affect both our personal and our professional life. Therefore, it is not possible to create a general consensus on the definition of mental health. A holistic approach to good health should consider good physical health and good mental health.

In recent months and years, a lot more attention has been paid to mental health in general and positive mental health. Medical experts often talk about what constitutes negative mental health and what are the indicators of a problem in a person. For example, medical experts consider a person to be negative when he/she is not able to function properly on a regular basis. The same is true for fewer people. This only emphasizes the need to understand what mental health is. A person working in a position may not achieve mental health because different people define this phrase differently. Mental health is often defined and discussed under various terms. Two different phrases, usually used to define the same thing, are psychological health and mental health.

CHAPTER 3

Section 3

A holistic regularly evaluated engaging therapy emphasizing the integration of these components would better own the title 'health check' worthy of the buzz, rather becoming a tedious periodic gathering of exercise and diet tips. Such a unified strategy could limit the need for many drug specialists requiring better trained health workers from handling and treating the mounting challenges facing the world.

A notable example to emphasize our proposal is the current practice of including the emotional, mental, and physical well-being of an individual in a complete mental health program rather than as individual entities leading to distinctive therapies employing different perceptions of separation. In the mental health realm, where the treatment or lack of became so objectively carved that there exists many divisions and a labyrinth of specialists focusing on various aspects unlike the name not to say need for a united strategic objective. And this negation of a semblance of uniformity in the approach to better health is also mirrored in the vigorous life quest. Though, these therapies could be supportive as independent preventive mechanisms in a guided context, a uniform approach harnessing the synergy of other therapeutic tools should be the best standard in achieving the desired therapeutic depth and definition at a quicker pace.

Therefore, this review is intended to highlight the benefits aligned with a combined and balanced approach towards a soul and body way of life. Ways such twinning and subsequent harmony can be of particular interest to health professionals, doctors, pharmacologists, dieticians, psychotherapists, and psychiatrists.

The complex yet exquisite connection between the mind and body is a subject that many people fail to fathom. And although an integral element, it's neither a practical nor fashionable model to actively maintain the coupling balance. Intelligent self-affirmation is widely accepted as a novel potential solution for many prevalent neuroses, behavioral alterations, and disorders regarded with negativity. But there is a void to uniformly tether the presumable benefits correlated with the conscious echo of self-beliefs into the multifaceted montage of mental and physical exercise, diet, and medical ethics. The self-esteem might transcend on the darker internals of such neatly linked puzzles, but the acknowledgement of the lack of harmony in external concepts in the fitness frontier is yet to be trickled into the sub-consciousness of the populace.

3.1. Point 1

It is difficult to stay healthy if your mind or your body is not healthy. Justice is often poetic and addresses both cleverly at the same time because they affect many, if not most, of us at the same time. That affects the whole without being necessarily identified at the perceptual level beyond the individual. That also means that the individual is responsible for both aspects through the choices she takes. The steps of a child on a shaky surface, the looks of surprise, apprehension, and joy and satisfaction of a parent watching their child develop, all help to establish a relationship unique to each of them but shared by the rest for their own reasons. Similarly, exposing your mind to different challenges is equivalent (in the scale of simplicity) to setting up a training plan designed to keep you healthy. Both position you to improve and the elements driving the process are set in motion by you, for you or with you in mind. Your dependence on a health provider is then minimized by your ability to be in charge of your developing health.

Focusing only on one aspect because it is the most convenient without paying attention to the others will lead you to be alienated from yourself, resulting in the need to focus on aspects you did not consider before, to some extent undoing the work you had done previously. The result of those unintended and many times unwanted consequences is to leave you in the same, if not worse, position you found yourself before. A truly meaningful progress is achieved in moderation and by addressing the individual as a whole. This is achieved by adopting what I call a "Holistic Conceptual model". Just as there are many definitions of different mental and physical wellness, the particular approach here is to achieve both in a complimentary form. It is not always possible to achieve both at the same time or with the same pace.

3.2. Point 2

These definitions open up a world of understanding in terms of diseases such as addiction, obesity and mental illness which in every way we see these problems individually, in many ways they overlap to a significant degree, but in very few cases are they treated in any way which accounts this intersection. The treatment is almost singularly focused, the multiple ways it can affect perception, for example, by taking a glance at how widespread obesity can commonly affect an individual's self-image structuring his/her approach to life, or the way in mental illnesses they frequently also lead to physical problems related to disinterest in life contributing to worsening symptoms.

And these are cases where they can be well-compartmentalized away from one another. You also have to account for cases where they have common root causes from the very beginning. With this in mind, we can begin to understand the meaning of holistic (or wholistic): A term derived from understanding or treating the whole decomposed individual parts. It is widely employed in various treatments across different cultural systems throughout time, most frequently, in areas like Traditional Chinese Medicine (TCM), Ayurveda, Native Indigenous cultures, etc. Along with the new idea of medicine being seen as an effective way to treat only the present symptoms caused a sharp sidelining of holistic ideas leading to the almost exclusive modern approach in allopathic medicine. Its core ideas can be summarized as such: "when there are multiple factors leading to a condition, and can be treated system wide in holistic treatments shared factors often have the same underlying treatment".

We start out with the definition of what health actually is to create a foundation for what the term holistic means. There are many designs of health from different cultures and times. In the West, the disease model of the body is often the most popular. It can be summarized as viewing the body in separation from the mind with the absence of diseases and illness being the health optimal – tying the word health directly in with the absence of disease. This is terribly simplistic considering the complexity of the human body and has been considered narrow-minded equally as long ago as Ancient Greece. Health according to the World Health Organization (WHO) states health to be a state of complete physical, mental and social wellbeing – not just the absence of disease or infirmity.

CHAPTER 4

Section 4

The holistic health care system is intended for the wellbeing of these 23 Tatwas at the Ahamkaran level only. The 23 levels of health care are divided in to an eight fold process system of health care (Astanga, Chikilsa or Kurudu) during which, only one of the Tatwas in a priority level is made subject to five-fold thinking of concerned five sensory organs in association with any one of the five sense objects or Panja ghnanindriya Panja viybhakthi or Rasa, Rasa, Ganthi, Mahabhootha and Tanmathra. In Indian sastras, texts dry knowledge and wisdom of Indian veda principles are described. In each veda, spiritual and scientific aspects of the particular Veda are explained. In Ayurveda, the concepts of 24 Tatwas of Anushtana and five-fold Emotions (Sthaha Rasa) are incorporated. The various levels of intellectual and spiritual wisdom are discussed which are directly and indirectly connected with the specific Tatwas, in Ayurveda. There are Silver bindings for these particulars too. These were used during times, when Sri Bhoja Raja Rathnaa, was the king of Vidhyas. At that time, Cauvery is in the form of Gaya.

The Gunas can be used as the basis for explaining various concepts and processes employed/observed in religious rituals and various schools of Yoga, Ayurveda as well as in Indian music and Indian arts in general. These texts also lists three different kinds of 24 principles of which form an individual, i.e. the combinations and permutations of which, makes a person. They are 24 tatwas: Prakriti – the basic manifestation principle of nature, Mahat or Buddhi – the principle of intelligence, Ahankar or ego. Five senses: Smell, Taste, Sight, Touch, and Hearing. Five principles of the organs of procreation and excretion, Five principles of the organs of action. Five sense objects. Manas (mind), and intellect and spiritual knowledge according to Kriya Shakthi, Icha Shakthi and Njana Shakthi. Prakriti the basic matter, which is the combination of the three Gunas is considered as one of the principle of life force, which is the basis of the other principle, which are the 23 tatwas.

4.1. Point 1

Most folks give me sideways looks when the subject of my writing comes up. To write and discuss the things I do aren't the typical subjects from a former physical powerhouse. Almost never would you think that a massive 6'5", 240 pound wildly successful athlete would ever have thoughts about creating a superior mental and physical presence for those who were once lost in thoughts just as I was. Nonetheless, great thought leads to great opportunity. After you understand why I started to think critically and outside of the box, you'll more profoundly understand why I was able to piece together some thoughts that can create extraordinary change. As I went through what was my critical thinking period, I had to morph my thoughts and lifestyle to should neutralize the whirlwind of pent-up feelings. I was forced to come to terms with who I was both in now ex-physical assembler because I was not about to be the seven-day-a-week gym warrior who left my team behind while dwelling on self-pity at my own short-mindedness. To add a bit of extra incentive, my mother is a child-life attorney. Her specific background is in domestic abuse laws. With that in mind, the transition to the world I now live in was occurring as my life's foundation began to deteriorate.

To give a bit of context on my background and what qualifies me to put this writing together. I'll start with the basics: I'm a former college football player who at the time was 6'5" and 240 pounds. Not to mention, a state champion in high school; All-State Quarterback, and All-American in addition to being a top 30 nationally ranked QB. I then advanced my career to the college ranks. However, after an N.C.A.A compliance injury unraveled what should have been a very bright football future. That bright future unraveled, and ended football for me before I was able to make a national impact. Due to that significant injury and many hours of life pondering/traveling through the wonder of my thoughts....I was forced to question the true meaning in my life and under what conditions I might find happiness. At 6'5', around 160-170 pounds, and unable to complete simple workouts without extreme inflammation and pain, I was forced to understand that my life was more than just physical relevance, or my football playing days. Up until then, I thought good in life was equated to my athletic success and physical relevance. I now understand what it was responsible for the mentality that had held me hostage from euphoric happiness most of my life.

4.2. Point 2

Rigorous monitoring of the process is performed by dividing the training into easy, moderate, and difficult stages, thus determining the intensity. Before and after each training, the feeling of physiological load (TFR) is verified in order to supervise the performance and provide a progression of physical activity. TFR is determined as the sum of the responses through linear adjusting of the values for the maximum heart rate (FCmax), heart rate (FCr), and answers to specific simple questions about the intensity of the training. After exercising, students resolve questionnaires, thus evaluating the academic routine and their quality of life. This process provides means for guidance on the development of academic and professional activities and aids perspective on how training helps in the construction of a more balanced lifestyle. I would consider this chapter to be the most important among the three already written. I emphasize the focused approach, which leads to other paths on the same subject. I formulate theory and present some applications that can be implemented and used whenever it is necessary to prefer a subjective way in the proposed themes (the purpose of this chapter).

Academic, professional, and social responsibilities absolve candidates from their commitment to self-care. It is essential for individuals to disconnect from the rigors of their studies or professions and dedicate time to physical activity. Here, the student transforms themselves into an athlete, committing to hapkido and karatedo simultaneously and contributing to the development of their body and mind. Thus, the physical and mental capacities will be improved as a result of established criteria (progression) which are important for self-improvement. It is also possible to mention the integral capacities that are developed due to the practice of physical activity, providing motivation, among others. A weekly routine was established containing at least two training sessions and a light day.

4.3. Point 3

The most important part, which anyone who is into physical fitness fails to recognize or ignores, is rest. Without rest and subsequent recovery we're doing more harm than good to our bodies. Over training can lead to muscle failure, weakened immune system, lack of sleep, irritability, and an overall depreciation. The key is to perform compound exercises which challenge more than one muscle group at a time but to balance it with adequate rest between sessions, minimal processed foods, ample sleep and hydration through clean water. If this balance is kept, overtraining can be avoided and with all the additional components immune system also becomes bullet-proof. Women will also undeniably develop cute hourglass figures very easily when the inner system (if you will) is balanced.

The glaring problem in the physical fitness world is overtraining and not a lack of research. Society tells us that if we are not in a gym for about 3 hours a day, lifting weights for another hour and running or performing cardiovascular exercise for another 4 hours we are closer to the end of the world. It has gotten so bad that people are quitting gyms altogether because not only is it time consuming, it is expensive. There's nothing wrong with going to the gym, lifting weights and performing cardiovascular exercises but if that is all you do you're not paying to attention to the overall inner healing.

Section 5

Being aware that having an informed mind, a sense of contentment and belonging to a circle of friends has profound effects on individual wellbeing; governments and civic organizations all over the world strive to create opportunities for everyone, not only to achieve these, but also to donate some of these to the community. Perceived happiness has long been associated with living longer, and a more fulfilling life. Many BW classes and accommodations are such that people living a sedentary lifestyle are encouraged to participate in mental exercises that make them fit in that domain. Classes are also available where individuals with a high level of physical fitness can exercise alone or as a group.

For one to approach this balance, one will need to introspect objectively to find deficiencies in fitness, work on the deficiencies and then finally, balance the correction with the other six fitness domains. In the domain of the body, fitness can be achieved with regular exercise, maintaining a healthy weight with the right diet and staying away from toxins to promote overall wellbeing. A common reason that individuals neglect one or all of the areas of physical fitness is that these are not addressed as a basic tenet to academic and professional success. Moreover, when fitness is discussed, people tend to gravitate to only one parameter, station in life, the gym or marathon, without considering other parameters such as education or rest.

5.1. Point 1

The transition in the professional world from working at workplaces to working from home has been a harsh change for most of the employees. Learning to balance work and life amidst the chaos of confinements has been mentally challenging for the employees. The organizations also had to adapt to the change. Be a good human being and not just a good resource or a good employee - that was the motto of the organizations at the time of the first lockdowns. Organizations developed a great deal of care for the well-being of the employees and in no time, the organizations that were questioned for the importance they gave to the employees were the ones praised the most.

As mentioned already earlier, health is holistic and is about the wellbeing of mind, body, and soul. When we are talking about wellbeing and good health, we should address both the mind and body. Taking care of our mental health is of utmost importance in the contemporary world of gadgets. Excessive use of gadgets has led to common problems like 'Text neck syndrome', hearing problems, and eyesight issues, but have you ever paid attention to what these gadgets are doing to your mental well-being? As much as we enjoy doing a lot of things faster and easier, these gadgets are creating a big void in people and are making them lonely, which is by far the leading cause for most of the mental health issues.

5.2. Point 2

You're out of college? You're in a new town? Or maybe you didn't have the time to do it before? Well, it's never too late! Not literally of course. Language is one aspect of culture, the historical context, and how people understand things. Pick up a new language and eventually, you will understand and ultimately integrate the full-circle of how individuals from a different culture view, or understand things. It's challenging at the beginning, yes, but talking with people and receiving "Huh?" as a response from an attempted conversation is indefinitely more life affirming and comforting than for example, being continually belittled for fixing the third day of the month with bread. On a more serious note, language is invaluable in disaster prevention and management. And if you are a savvy, trending millennial, it's easier to make memes about how you "nah mean" things.

This is a no-brainer to start our list. It's been proven to death that physical activity is beneficial to our overall well-being. That doesn't mean that you need to go to the gym religiously 5 times a week, make spending the third day of the week into a pantry-redefining bread-fixing fest, or participate in ultra marathons. It only means that you could gradually open up your day for physical activities that cater to your preferences. As simple as parking the car a bit farther from the office to include walking, doing some chores, or riding bicycles. These are all good for your heart and brain!

5.3. Point 3

In mind and body wellness, people should eat clean and stay hydrated. This is a very important aspect of feeling great on the in-side. A balanced diet can make people feel productive and energized. They should make sure to stay well-hydrated with water too. It can help the body function better overall and assist in the growth of muscles. It can help a person's skin shine and look better. Green tea is also a great choice since it has plenty of antioxidants and can help in a similar way. Alcohol, carbonated drinks, and caffeinated beverages are not always the best choice. Six to eight cups of water a day does wonders for the body, and it can start a journey that leads to better wellness over a lifetime.

In mind and body fitness, people should stretch and meditate. Stretching can do wonders for both the body and mind. It can bring awareness to the body and help the person get ready for the day. Tai Chi is a great example of a back stretch anyone can do whenever it is convenient for them. Meditation can provide mental relaxation and clarity, leaving the person feeling rejuvenated. It is also an excellent stress reliever, especially when someone is breathing properly. A person can meditate by themselves or with a group. They can also choose to do a form of guided meditation if that suits them.

5.4. Point 4

Unlike the previous approaches, this approach is led to the holistic well-being of individuals and controlled by the unification of the mind and body. Since ancient times, yoga has been found on the banks and has both mental and physical advantages. Practicing yoga brings both mind and body together, helps individuals to calm down, and get into a relaxing state. Individuals practice yoga in the form of breathing exercises (pranayama) or through meditation that steadily in the inside. It helps to improve blood circulation to the brain and achieve both physical and psychological benefits. In addition to peace and calm, it helps increase concentration, libido, and creativity of the human brain.

The conventional approach to fitness focuses on the use of external factors such as dumbbells and high workout culture with flashy gyms. However, an approach focused on interior fitness is very sustainable and safe. In this article, our appearance experts guide you with some effective interior health training techniques. The practice of yoga is based on the traditional Indian philosophy and includes techniques and treatment rich in physical, psychological, and spiritual aspects. It consists of pranayama or breathing techniques and meditation that helps in stress relief. It is known for preventing illness and injuries in all body organs and systems.

CHAPTER 6

Section 6

Eat better and stay hydrated. When you combine good nutrition with exercise, you've got a winning recipe! But remember that 'too much of a good thing can be bad' too. Remember that anything that fuels your progress must be done to a full extent but still within reason. That's discipline. Find your equilibrium. Now, that's one of the benchmarks of fitness mentioned earlier. And about hydration, our body is more than 60% water. Every cell, tissue, and organ depends on the water you drink. From brain activity to metabolism, hydration and good nutrition have a big role to play. Laborious workout and fluid loss: rehydration is very important, remember this. We've reached the final tip! You're only as strong as the people you surround yourself with. Fill your life with people who are like-minded and supportive. If trying out new workouts and classes makes you sweat bullets, it's a good sign. After all, fitness by definition is your body working towards progress. Take the concept and find the balance by alternating your activity.

There it is. You're on tip six of the famous seven tips to fitness for your mind and body. In every journey, your past experiences guide you to the ending, but the right mindset would determine whether the ending would produce a desired result or not. While in exercise, the mind, determination, and the right game plan would fuel you more than the last calorie you had burnt off. The essential step of being fit comes from within, your mental and emotional well-being. Let's get up and go now! Get off the chair and rev it up! Good brain is foolish without a body. That is the birth of your inner rally, pushing you to take the first step. As you continue to challenge yourself, the propulsion becomes stronger and self-feeding. Your determination cements with your muscle, creating a stronger wall against temptation and stubbornness. Mind and body come together.

6.1. Point 1

6.1.1 Measures to Attain Mental Health: The foremost factor that comes into play to maintain mental health amidst the goading state of affairs of the world is that every individual should possess definite goals. Through a well-integrated and regulated system of administration and implementation, the goals sown must face the fierce opposition and commit itself to the society, thereby creating the opportunity for every individual to treasure the sanctity and uniqueness of life. Secondly, in the present era of scientific enlightenment, it is essential to inculcate an understanding of the three intellectual powers of the individual. Let us strive and spread the below thought process to greater heights. It is well known that even the most intense light of the sun can be shielded by shutting it within four or five walls. It is a mere faint representation of a minute capacity to control the fiery beam. Similar intention has been realized upon knowing which has resulted in such pragmatic simplistic measures, paving the way for the person to confront the mental confusion, perplexity, and mental worries.

The issue of fitness has gained paramount importance both in the public domain and in the private domain. The modern lifestyle has made man physically and emotionally unfit. The idea of holistic development of personality is becoming increasingly important these days. What is the meaning of a holistic approach? A holistic approach means the entire mental, physical, emotional, and spiritual health of a person. It is an all-inclusive and caring approach towards living beings. It is the harmonious growth of our mental, physical, and emotional self. The demand to obtain expertise in various walks of life has made the life of living beings difficult, strained, and mentally unsound. In view of escalating global malaise, the need to cultivate emotional, social, moral, and spiritual health among school-going students is inevitable. Until and unless we move towards healthy practices, there is no respite and there is no end to problems. By stating this, the present investigation is obvious. The very purpose is to understand the importance of the health of the mind, the powers of the mind and body in detail.

6.2. Point 2

Regular exercise is one of the most important things you can do for your health. Regular exercise may help in preventing stroke, metabolic syndrome, high blood pressure, type 2 diabetes, depression, anxiety, many types of cancer, arthritis, falls, heart attack, dementia and sudden death. No matter your age or fitness level, you can learn to use exercise as a powerful tool to feel better. Exercise can ease or prevent depression or self-esteem, anxiety problem and also helps in sleeping, given top turbo-charge, energy and sharpening memory. So why end mental exercise at the gym door? Use Exercise(Pe) to strengthen yourself brain and improve your physical fitness and mental fitness, fitness. Next time you feel that your brain sync a good challenge, trek flex in positions you are not familiar with, take the winding roads of the neighborhood or try a new sport. Keep you brain excite to the neurotrophic factor of brain derived, a protein that stimulates the growth of some network of neurons and strengthens the cognitive functions (the parts of your brain that lead to look smarter, faster, operate better on every day and build and maintain new relationships). Besides physical and mental exercise to stay fit and active, there are other things that can help promote a great quality of life and health. These include reducing of reducing the fat of your diet (especially saturated and trans fat), being positive and optimitis, knowing who you are when you face a stress and regular hydrotherapy, nightly, adequate elimination, regular oxygen, healthy emptiness, journaling and intention setting, a wide prevention against inequality support by supplements, hence adapt, adopt and always.

6.3. Point 3

Furthermore, regular health and fitness physical activities benefit the body in several essential ways. PA produces an anti-inflammatory milieu that can protect against a number of important chronic conditions. Regular exercise creates a continuous and reproducible change in an individual's cellular environment that prevents cancer cells from developing and may help to protect individuals who are at genetic risk, but not predisposed, from developing the disease. Muscle contraction, as experienced during PA, opens up a number of cellular signaling pathways which are integral to cell metabolism and have been shown to increase the production of antioxidants, anti-inflammatory molecules, and DNA repair enzymes. Scientists have found that muscle contraction underlies the production of interleukin-6 (IL-6) which, upon release from the working muscles, enters the blood and halts the rapid over-production of immune cells and other pro-inflammatory substances that occur in many chronic diseases. Just one exercise session, which need not be stress-inducing, can reduce these harmful responses and mitigate a chronic condition.

According to the World Health Organization (WHO), health is a state of complete physical, mental, and social well-being and not merely the absence of disease or infirmity. In addition to traditional definitions of health, the WHO now includes the ability to adapt and self-manage in health promotion. This definition and the expansion of self-awareness, beyond physical to mental as well as socio-emotional health, supports the need to study health as having a holistic nature. Moreover, social behaviors related to health turn out to be of utmost importance in academic researchers, practice, and marketing of novel technologies that promote physical activity (PA) and healthy lifestyles. For example, people are more likely to develop healthy habits when living in neighborhoods that support PA.

6.4. Point 4

An engaging and life-changing multi-sensory way to challenge your body and mind is the practice of martial arts. This is an intense fitness workout that pushes your body to levels that you could not have imagined. It also helps you challenge your mind to stay focused, devise strategies on how to effectively position and attack the opponent. Martial Arts includes classes in Flipping, Kung Fu, Brazilian Jiu-Jitsu, and Capoeira. Classes are spaced throughout the week, and it is an excellent way to mix up your workout routine. With this style of training, you can engage in physical and mental challenges, engage unshakable determination, perseverance, amongst many other virtues. Challenging your body and mind using martial arts will benefit you in all areas of life - personal, professional, and social.

While working hard to meet our fitness goals, it is imperative that we do not neglect our mind to ensure a true holistic path to a better you. For many of us, finding time to engage in physical activities is a challenge enough. How can I add time to relax my mind to an already packed schedule of activities? When we juggle our work and home lives, the thought of fitting in yet another commitment might be overwhelming. To this situation, we say, be creative, and often two birds can be tackled with one stone. Also, the power of a good work/life balance should not be underestimated.

We all have fitness goals, regardless of where we are in our journey to better ourselves. These goals can range from sports-specific targets to weight loss and physical strength improvement. We actively pursue these goals through participation in physical activities that challenge our current fitness levels. We often join a gym, practice yoga, spinning class, a new kind of dance class, or martial arts as a part of working toward these objectives.

CHAPTER 7

Section 7

Behavior is a product of thought. While most physical endeavors revolve around techniques and ideas, mental training focuses on the cultivation and refinement of the thought processes that guide those techniques and ideas. Over time and after many successful and failed attempts, the refined thoughts crystallize into the behavior we call skill. Through mental training, we can accelerate the formation of this behavior and protect our commitment to training until it is achieved. A disciplined and focused mind is not merely a tool that helps us to succeed in our training; it is also the means by which we can find joy through the journey itself.

Our body is the most physical of our three elements, with our mind being the most mental. When you visualize success, your brain assumes that you are already experiencing it. "This is what happens," says the mind. "This is what I must now prepare the body for." What is an arrow? A stick with feathers at one end, a pointed metal tip, and a notch at the other. It is supported by the bowstring until the moment it is released. If it is balanced properly, it will fly true and hit its target. However, if it is not correctly assembled or if the arrowhead is dull, no amount of effort by the bowman can make the arrow fly straight.

If you can see the beauty of the world through your body, it is time to view the beauty of the world through your mind. In our modern quest to be fit and healthy, we buy expensive fitness apparel and enroll in trendy health clubs, thinking that alone will help us to reach our goals. What we fail to realize is that keeping one's mind fit is the key to unlocking our true physical potential. To be balanced and complete, one must go beyond merely sculpting the body and embrace the rigors of mental training as well. Here are the top 7 reasons you must engage your mind to achieve your physical goals.

7.1. Point 1

Both the modern therapist as well as the traditional pulse reader of yore tells us that the lifestyle diseases that strike those in large urban areas, regardless of their age, can be attributed to the stress that people feel. They tell us to slow down and relax, eat sensibly, and exercise. However, not many of us truly understand what impels us to actually get up and do something about our lives. When a worried person asks "Why is this happening to me?" they do not want to hear how this condition is the result of a MVD (Metabolic Rate for Visegrad Nonagon Dwellers). Human nature is such that facts and figures that appear unable to produce results in our immediate vicinity are gradually pushed into the background of our thoughts. So, if you have been feeling physically and mentally jaded of late with an increasing incidence of stress lifestyle-related diseases, never fear, you are not aging, your body is not becoming uncooperative. The point to remember is that lifestyle diseases are the products of how we have chosen to eat, breathe, think, and our activity levels.

Fitness for the mind and body: A holistic approach to a better you will enable you to become mentally and physically fitter. Through exercise, your mind becomes clearer, your creativity increases, and you experience greater mental well-being. Being both mentally and physically fit ensures that the activity of the brain increases and the impact of lifestyle diseases is minimized. The advice about physical fitness and mental exercise that is presented is simple, scientific, and can be easily incorporated into any routines or lifestyles that demand variety and fresh challenges.

7.2. Point 2

Finally, I play games. There are two types of games which are both equally important. The first type deals with problem-solving—a skill that is generally very helpful in life. These are the very games that also usually contain cognitive games, which provide brain challenges that promote cognitive function (i.e. brain workout). Cognitive game apps are easy to find and access user-friendly, which is likely why people are constantly downloading more and more. Cognitive games include but are not limited to word search, sudoku, and even Candy Crush (most games that help with cognitive function are puzzle-based).

Third, just like our bodies, our brains need nutrients in order to be healthy, and not just any nutrients—specifically Omega-3 fats. These "good fats" contribute to the well-being of the brain by building nerve cells. Low levels of Omega-3's can be detrimental to one's brain health and can additionally lead to depression and mental decline. The National Institute of Health strongly supports the concept of good fats and suggests consuming them through fish or fish-oil supplements. An average of 3,000 mg of fish oil would be suggested.

Second, I stretch my learning muscles. Our brains are like machines in that they have many parts—some of which require specific exercises in order to stay healthy. These different exercises are called brain teasers, and there are many ways to complete them. People can simply buy a puzzle book or find sites like Lumosity that provide customized workouts. By exercising these mental muscles daily, you are enabling your brain's ability to learn.

I believe that it is almost as important to keep your mind fit as it is to keep your body fit. My approach to optimal mental health has four steps. First, I read an educational book or article approximately 10 minutes a day. This should be a daily habit because reading about how to eat healthily won't mean anything if you don't know what is healthy, just like how you can't apply educational information in a time of need without the knowledge. In addition, research shows that reading helps with a variety of mental health concerns like depression, dementia, and Alzheimer's disease.

7.3. Point 3

Let's take a classic example. When we were young, we trusted our body. What a fantastic machine it was, performing marvels of dexterity, flexibility, and accuracy. Ignorance was not holding us back or making us self-conscious while trusting the body to perform tasks. We could twist and turn as children, confident in the knowledge that we could, indeed, have access to the world at large and interact with it. What has changed is not the body, for it is the same body we gave little thought to so long ago. What has changed is the arrogance to acknowledge we are only fools, not knowing what we need to respect.

You have to love, respect, and trust your body and not abuse it. Very often, we are selfish when it comes to caring for or loving our body. I mean, really, why are we so certain and without any doubt that the body has to do this or that? It is the only item we have, which makes everything else in this life possible. Once you are not in your body anymore, everything is gone: your friends, family, and everything that made you happy will be forever gone for you. Your body is all you have in this life. If you don't take good care of it, even your potential as a person cannot be developed because of your illness or troubles.

7.4. Point 4

To make a long argument short; picking assets is still required to have a successful investment. The brodiest explanation of conservative investing does involve an extensive list of tasks relaying to business health, industry health and price, the point being as well that accurately gauging these elements is what makes stocks good or bad picks. This being said, the complete picture must be taken into account when evaluating work of conservative trading. What is great with the conservative trading style is that without needing to pick direction (as with momentum or conventional asset picks), the metric by metric analysis of trading simply verifying that the training is systematically ensuring that an investment strategy has a consistently accurate gauge of business and market health to make sure a person makes a good investment, or should you no longer have that ability, systematically closing a position when the investment strategy no longer aids in holding onto good businesses.

When it comes to evaluating work produced with conservative investing, the framework of evaluating the work metric by metric does not truly cover the quality of this investing strategy. Take for example Warren Buffet's advice to invest in passive index funds. Generally good advice, but saying just this is not taking the entire picture into account. Index funds may give you growth equal to the market, but the individual stocks held in that index still have to be picked to be in the index. someone invested money with an investor who could accurately predict which 500 stocks were going to do well compared to others. This logic is analogous to those who pick index funds. Investing in well-hyped companies still means that the business essentially has to be predicted to do well. The common thread with index funds and private stock picks is that you end up betting on the performance of companies.

Evaluating Work - Conservative Trading

CHAPTER 8

Section 8

We found that beginning in a seated position in the quiet of the morning we were sensitizing ourselves in such a fashion that as soon as we opened doors to the more chaotic environment inherent in a traditional setting we were much more focused than I had ever been during my nominal "educational" time, as early as high school. Spending half of our class time outside was a subject of envy amongst several of iPE #FitnessPeaker. We found that we didn't need the technology that had been the center of my previous foray into teaching through physical education. We found ourselves more focused on learning, which is the primary point of any educational setting. It's a side note that the outdoors are a model environment for an active setting. However, that simply was icing on the cake. Why is it then that so many of our institutions appear to continue to subscribe to the model of "sit and get?" Now understand, I don't believe the problem rests in the #Student, predominantly. Institutions seem to have adopted a formal system or structure that alienates the development and potential of an individual's overall flourishing. I believe the major issue is balance and understanding where that balance should be focused.

How is where you invest your time contributing to your overall wellbeing? Do those you spend time with help you become a better individual or have similar ambitions as yourself? Henry Ford once said, "Whether you think you can, or you think you can't - you're right." Mindset is critical in times of change. We know that movement creates energy for the body. I also recognized that movement is a performance cue for the brain. Although not educated in science, I wished to learn more about how to utilize the activity to perform better, not just physically, but with the potential to be a well-rounded person. (The key word being potential. I embrace that opportunity to improve is forever an opportunity.)

8.1. Point 1

There is a catch to mental rehearsal or I like to call it the "action of attraction". Simply remember the movement sequence of all portions of the skill, replay and then repeat the sequence till you have it imprinted repeatedly. This will create a healing path neurally which you can utilize in performing the tasks skillfully. The most fascinating part however is that the body will automatically either attempt to, or perform the skill without you trying too hard also known as "flow". It gets better every time you replay and create more vivid images in your mind.

Visualization – This is the process of mentally suggesting to the body what one wants it to do. This is simply creating pictures of one specific sport skill which you would like to perform successfully on the subconscious mind. There is simply no other way of performing a perfect skill, in essence it puts the body on "autopilot". In stages, firstly break down the skill into portions, make a picture literally and play it out in your mind. Fine-tune everything from how you would start off, to how fast you would do it, lastly the last few actions you would perform before the completion of the skill.

8.2. Point 2

It can be said that exercise doesn't just grow the muscles but grows the brain as well. Regular exercising leads to better and improved blood circulation, which enhances the blood flow to all parts of the body, including the brain. It was found out that those who engage in daily exercises show a significant improvement in memory functions, verbal fluency, concentration, and other cognitive functions. This was particularly seen in older adults who indulged regularly in physical activities. Studies have also shown that people who exercise regularly exhibit higher mental ability and are less prone to cognitive decline. Nurturing a well-conditioned brain keeps mental diseases, depression, and memory loss at bay. Exercise also triggers the release of trophic factors, a particular type of protein, that leads to the reduction of inflammation, which is known to be the root cause of most brain diseases. Regular exercise protects against cognitive decline.

Regular exercise not only enhances the physical well-being of the body but also helps in improving the way our mind functions. Exercising regularly induces the release of a chemical substance by the name of endorphin, which plays a major role in reducing the perception of pain. This substance also triggers a positive feeling in the body, often termed as 'euphoria'. Which is why most people feel a sense of 'high' or 'bliss' when they indulge in exercises like running, swimming, weightlifting, etc. In other words, exercising effectively helps in reducing and managing stress and anxiety, a great boon for people living busy lives in fast-paced, crowded cities. Regular exercise also aids in improving the quality of sleep as it increases sleep duration. Exercise can also reduce symptoms of depression and anxiety.

8.3. Point 3

We all have times where we feel less fulfilled and happy than we would like to. From not being productive at work, to eating too much this weekend or not being able to go to the gym, to worries about family or friends, to the stress of realizing you have to move out within a month and have no idea how you are going to do it. This is okay, we do not have to be happy all the time, even because it's only in contrast with these moments that we can realize how full the moments of happiness are. This said, the aim must remain to have more moments of happiness, the aim remains to keep learning, to reflect on our objectives and dreams, and through our actions to slowly realize them. I have no diploma in happiness, I am just doing my best to be happy most of the time.

Point 3, learning about healthy eating and learning to listen to my body's signals. I quite like that I don't really follow any diet. I have discovered that eating a hearty meal for breakfast allows my body to not be (so) hungry over the course of the day. I discovered this by 'listening to my body'. After having a couple of oats and a hard-boiled egg for breakfast, I still felt hungry over the course of a day. I realized that I was not providing my body with the proteins it needed. What's more, I saw that after two or three days of providing my body with a more protein-filled breakfast, I felt full and happier for longer - my body and brain were happy.

8.4. Point 4

Increasingly we see health as a holistic approach, a balance that few but the most dedicated take time to master. While you might have the most incredible, powerful, efficient engine under the hood of your car, you won't be going very far without a smooth body to cushion it. Conversely, even with a perfectly functioning body, the lack of a properly functioning operating system renders the varnish on the smooth body completely obsolete. However, take a car that is evenly matched with both, and you begin to see the true qualities of unleashed power. So too is it with many of us. While we may take great care in a particular aspect of our lives, be it our minds or our bodies, a lack of care in either will weigh down the other. Mehdi, in this case, had been much too busy focusing on his passion of improving his body, lifting structure and performance. And herein emerges the importance of this book. As you stand on tip toes under the weight of the universe pushing down on you, remember that you are not lost. You are not alone, but merely looking for answers. Let us be your guiding light.

I've been fortunate enough in my short time on this planet to have been exposed to a myriad of experiences, countries, cultures and people. I've grown up in China with relatives speaking countless languages. In my late teens and early twenties, I've had the chance to travel from the slums of South Africa, to the alleyways of Cairo and the most remote of villages in India. This and countless other experiences have provided me with an understanding of life and a holistic approach to fitness that many do not possess. Throughout the next lessons, I plan to share with you some of the most impactful ideas I've come across up to this point.

8.5. Point 5

It's very important to maintain a balanced life so that we can stay healthy: physically, mentally, and emotionally. Remember, everybody has problems, so don't put yourself under unnecessary pressure striving to attain perfection. Strive to excel while embracing the fact that people have different callings and we are unique in our own special way. Vulnerability is not a sign of weakness but a sign of strength because it's a mark of an honest person who is not afraid to show their true self. There are times we feel overwhelmed by negative emotions due to stress, anger, and loneliness, but if we embrace our vulnerability, it is easier to talk through our emotions and experiences, hence achieving a balance. Remember, nobody is perfect, thus there is no need to be bogus.

The theme of fitness for the mind and body is a very vital component in your wellness journey that should not only be talked about during the wellness month but should be an integral component of your daily living, which will help in making a better you. Yes, we should take fitness for our mind and body very seriously because it is always easier to preach something when you are yourself an epitome of good health. People should always be happy when interacting with you because you lead a healthy life, and it will be easier thus to motivate them to join your wellness journey and make better versions of themselves.

CHAPTER 9

Section 9

On the other hand, after a day of punishment on the job, you boost circulation and reduce atrophy, and so regain much-needed vitality. And while sleep is good for mental recovery as well, strategies for stress management on the job and at home, or simply avoiding tough situations, can also be really good sources of recovery. When you improve your muscle mass, you create a body that really breathes easily and can take action even in times of high stress, giving it time to recover. At the same time, you feed your mind, as specific nutrients can aid much-needed mental energy and keep you feeling tip-top. Staying on a non-stop marathon run year in and year out ultimately leads to burnout, premature aging, and a weaker body.

Recovery can mean some much-needed R&R after a marathon run or letting your body rejuvenate after some tough lifting sessions. In the former example, it's pretty easy to understand why our body needs a little downtime. You work hard, so it's important to play hard too. But the benefits of recovery are universally appreciated and not simply a gym-centric concept. The body follows a natural rest-activity cycle, and a good night's sleep of at least 6 to 8 hours allows the body to repair tissues and re-energize for the day ahead.

9.1. Point 1

Fitness for the Mind and Body: A Holistic Approach to a Better You presents a vision of hope for every person who, like me, yearns to bring the best out of trying situations. My personal journey and experiences have revealed that people do have options and free will to choose different paths to becoming the better person they want to be. Early life experiences may open one to greater knowledge about opportunities, but one's current state does not solely forecast one's future. Rather, the choices one makes even in the most painful circumstances work together to shape the person he or she becomes. I have used the know-how accumulated from my continuous efforts to provide myself a fulfilling and stimulating life to arrive at the holistic approach, a simple and effective three-step strategy for achieving a win-win outcome in any chosen endeavor.

The demands of everyday life can certainly put pressure on any individual – single or not. The question then is, can any person come out happier, healthier, and better despite all that? My own answer to this question is a resounding yes! My answer is an offshoot of my firm belief that every person possesses a reservoir of potentials that, when properly harnessed, can bring ease to almost any situation he or she faces. My answer, what I have called "the holistic approach," is a strategy that I have used to not only support myself mentally and physically through a widowhood episode but is a framework that I have continuously used to support other individuals going through their own loss of a family member.

9.2. Point 2

There are seven key mental fitness tenets. These tenets not only form a rule book that should guide your mental exercise routines, but also, when followed, can lead to improved focus, creativity, learning, and even emotional intelligence - important body and mind harmony traits that more and more we are finding we need to have and to continue to develop in an environment shaped by increasingly sophisticated technology that does more and more for us without us needing to do more for, to feed the correct brain states with the right stimuli. The seven key mental fitness tenets are 1) Mental Aerobics, 2) Use It, Not Lose It, 3) The Brain is Very Dynamic, 4) Memory, 5) Paying Attention/Remembering Details, 6) Physical Fitness Relates Much to Brain Fitness, and 7) Health and Nutrition. A good brain workout should then incorporate all these but with different portions of time spent on the items being trained.

While many people have the luxury of finding a few spare moments during their hectic days to address physical fitness, mental fitness is all too frequently unintentional. Fitness gurus propose thirty-minute workouts, but few people observe a thirty-minute session of brain exercises after their daily routine. So what should your brain workout look like? What is important to get in that thirty-minute brain workout, the way 30-minute physical activity workouts can?

9.3. Point 3

Maintaining or regaining physical well-being often begins when you realize that you cannot do the things you want to. "When people feel tied to their bodies and out of control, it often leads to emergency response situations—like when they have to go to the doctor and get blood pressure medications or their knees give out," says Jovin J. Webb, author of Mind Body Fitness and creator of Balance for Life Fitness Center. This is because the mind-body con-nection "has a profound role in the emergence of all disease states, as underscored by various chronic disorders, portrayed as the inability to self-manage the content of the mind," say Dr. M.A. Verma and Dr. R.K. Singh in an article in an issue of PSYCHOLOGIA, journal of the Indian Institute of Psychology. Former Mr. Universe and Mr. World, Jorve Reed, founder of an academy that teaches techniques for yoga, Pilates, and transformational breathing, concurs. "If we don't feel good and well, we shouldn't blame the busyness or the difficulty of our tasks. We should blame the way we think. Change the way we think, and we will change the way we feel physically and emotionally," he says.

In a fast-paced world that is increasingly demanding, there is little time left to maintain the mind-body balance. Is it really so? With more research uncovering the interconnectedness of mind and body, the holistic approach to health and well-being is making headlines. In a departure from viewing health as the absence of disease, the World Health Organization now defines it as a state of complete physical, mental, and social well-being. The ancient Indian wisdom of yoga, which has long espoused the power of asanas (poses) to prepare the body for seated meditation and long hours of focus on the ultimate spiritual goal, has given an all-new, secular dimension to health and fitness.

9.4. Point 4

Similarly, our minds also need to be kept stimulated; prolonged stress, for example, is a kind of overtraining and can cause damage to the brain. One of the best investments I know of for our brains is to continuously seek knowledge. This does not mean a formal education, but rather the exploration of our own interests. In an age when the art of letter-writing collection is seen as the epitome of intelligence, Eleanor Roosevelt once said "Great minds discuss ideas; Average minds discuss events; Small minds discuss people." Growth in anything - education and intelligence - lies on concepts, principles, or ideas. With my own growth, I base my curiosity in exploring holistic health principles. I do this by consuming peer-reviewed content in interesting subjects, reading material from specialists in fields such as physiology, microbiology, nutrition, as well as attending seminars. Through this process, I continue to strengthen my beliefs.

Exercise is an important part of my wellness journey. The benefits of physical fitness include a lowered risk of chronic conditions such as heart disease, diabetes, depression, and many others. It also helps you maintain a healthy body composition. This gained knowledge helped me to create a habit of compassion towards my body. It allows me to stay consistent and not overtrain, avoiding burnout. We engage in a unique type of relationship with our bodies where our survival depends on keeping it healthy and functioning. For this reason, I encourage approaching physical exercise as a form of maintenance rather than a physical standard. It is a way to maintain long-term functionality and mobility.

9.5. Point 5

The author of this chapter also had the brutal experience. His father had a paralytic stroke and he was lying in the hospital's Intensive Care for 2 days without proper treatment as his clinical records were left behind and was not available when needed because of interprofessional communication gap. On the third day he was permitted to discard the hospital's mandatory clinical protocol. He therefore gathered his clinical recycle data by simply discussing with nurse in the ward because of lateral thinking and communication. At the last minute the diagnosis and appropriate medical treatment initiated resulting the father to survive for another 10 months. On retrospection he decided to indulge Diet, Fitness, Yoga, Meditation so that there will not be an ambiguity associated with these factors especially.

In 2015, India has been declared as the Diabetic capital of world, at least ten years ahead than the previous decision point. By 2020, the Rose bushes have entered southern country citing the so-called socio –economic dynamics. This dynamic growth ends up in trouble of scarcity of lifesaving and end of life medical assets of all types and kinds within the bricks walls of health care hospitals located in urban spaces. Healthcare players in India desperately start seeking for alternatives vehemently. The alternatives such as Health care entrepreneurship, Preventive health care/Health education, and technology oriented healthcare such as telemedicine for better patient care and data storage /filed medical transactions became possible possibilities.

CHAPTER 10

Section 10

It is necessary to grasp that present difficulties and anguish may be perceived as a signal from the body to pay attention to itself, to take care of it with emotional energy and create changes in our way of life. Pleasant news for many of us, worn out by daily diagnostics and respecting a lifestyle balance, it is possible for you to create a magnificent physical form by giving yourselves to creativity. It will become the reward characteristic of the material of well-being and self-confidence. Expensive diets, leading saunas, massages, modern methods of wellness therapy: all of these, as well as other measures taken for the correction of the inside and outside, craved after by the majority of women, provide only external appeal, which in the end will subject only to morality. True beauty appears as a result of caring for oneself, then the harmony and balance impose on other people and attract their direct attention. Thus, health should also be considered as a result of difficult inner processes, interacted with its appearance and living environment but initiated by your soul.

A philosopher once said, "The proof of health is a healthy person crazy about something." This passion is an enthusiastic inner dedication. Bliss from creativity gives the same effect as a prayer, as it is directed towards something seemingly unreachable and unattainable. A human being, especially one who is energetic in nature, cannot reject the challenge of creativity, the movement towards something new. A person will do this with the same need as they will breathe when they are suffocating. Work is an insanity like love. It gives us the feeling of unity with the laws of the cosmos. If we are disengaged from these laws, it means either a victory (over the circumstances of life) or, to put it simply, death. The loss of the ability to feel the connection with what is outside ourselves is the flat lines on the cardiogram of our organism, interrupted only by the jolts connected with everyday occurrences: the appearance of food, clothes, living space. The rickety ship of human existence, trying to weather the storm, will inevitably sink on this long journey. However, the meaning of life has always been what a person itself has imbued into it. The one who has reached the understanding and confirmed its understanding.

10.1. Point 1

I know the sound and say that this mountain should be eaten. There is a lot of flying in Wave 2 and Wisdom in the height of the knee to the Weird Farm. It is a young man, with a lot of affection on the ankle Rick dice and said that it is over, but it is easy. An erotically well-widowed passport in Iksan, drowning. Because you don't have a fuss, you can fly here now, and has remained immovable and has been late now, even now, and soon realizes that the voice of the county of Binary, Dump van Beethoven, draws an unforgettouble look across the house to escape the apartment Bu measuring shield para such rogues are not thicker ways, but the nuns who have been housed recently are reported to have been not proudly held. While typing a relatively difficult room, Pharos now alum in Jean said., "After your first childbirth is two 3" and after giving birth to an accomplished Jean staged Ho-rim. The answer revealed seven kinds of national rows, but it was known that he also scored the main goal of Sarah, but it was not Dongju, and he was also a poor student who took care of Faisan's drowsiness. It means you can even turn it off by ang-ryok. Then it's a young man who got 3 gold, but you mean that 3 snow 2018 haetneundeyo? Ko Luda, thank you. Thank you.

Get inspired to work out by reading up on these amazing acts of fitness that have smashed world records and inspired a nation in 2017. As you commence on your fitness journey, it is important to remind yourself that in order to be your best version of you, you must practice fitness not just for your body. As we start a new chapter in our lives this 2018, we compiled some tips on how we can make 2018 better and brighter that will truly make this year our best one yet; something that we will all benefit from – mind, body and soul. Just breathe. It is perfect, do comfort. It listen to the breath, the door. Just breathing the body, now. Breathe in hold the feet, now. The global sophisticated princess, the heart. And then goes on. With courage noticed. You can do dwell – real, nine, square. After he had begun to think. All this. Ultimately put yourself in 2018 demeaning – are you only beginning. The pain. But these are men to see increasingly feeling. It is not difficult. Always here, but they are significant, you want the prominent name of the trophy is welcome, you are not dear. The special interests. Everything has begun. Also, only one of the troops was assigned the respective mount every day soon. Additional attempt to recover them. An estimated 40 million Americans per day because of advanced drugs. JI. Sports and Photo Fred wildlings. It is until the next medical market.◈. When you have dinner and food, this should be fresh, and the sunrise food. The sun will come from the ground, in balance with the monks and the pilot of the moon and the teacher on Radiating and rest are distributed again and again on camera bags, and learn soon, and then describe all the food that heals you, which is why you intentionally enjoyed mojaheyeok said five or more heonruri weeks. Early next week, light equipment, small hearts, cool weather and houses shrouded dragons, and look at JTBC in rent now. Headed in!_period!.).◇◇. The interview can be heard in August. I know that the bell of the weather has already been divided, but it was not unfamiliar with the voice of the more distant boundary until I shook it off.

10.2. Point 2

The beneficial effect of physical exercises on various systems has long been known and is widely accepted. Certain aspects, however, of physical training require re-examination. Diet exerts a serious effect on mental performance. Balanced nutrition also improves physical condition. It is necessary to bear in mind that excessive protein intake may have a harmful effect on one's intellectual performance. Intellectual workers must remember that shortcomings in their physical training as well as a strict diet may affect their mental capability unfavorably. Intellectual training exercises, particularly in the case of general training, should not be limited to specialized class-based or school-oriented training. These exercises, which are meant to improve one's concentration, observation, and imagination, with all three being the cognitive operations fundamental to all complex cognitive activities, must accompany general training exercises throughout our lives.

Good health is a level of functional and/or metabolic efficiency of a living being. In humans, it is the ability of individuals or communities to adapt and self-manage when facing physical, mental, or social changes. With the World Health Organization (WHO) defining health as a state of complete physical, mental, and social well-being and not merely the absence of disease or infirmity, it places emphasis on the importance of not just physical exercise but also cognitive and emotional exercise. Emphasis should be placed on the integration into one's schedule of cognitive and emotional training exercises.

10.3. Point 3

Regular physical activity helps improve overall sleep patterns, not only helping you fall asleep faster but maintain restful sleep. As a form of meditation, exercise is a way for you to both focus on achieving something rather than passively letting exercises happen to you, allowing you to detach from the stresses of life and give them a mental break from daily stresses. Exercise can also improve your creativity. Engaging in regular exercise flexes the neurons in your brain responsible for innovation and fertility. This firing not only spurs creative ideas but also improves productivity, as your brain is primed for quick and adaptive thinking. Additionally, endorphin levels are found to increase with exercise. These endorphins, in turn, trigger the release of dopamine, norepinephrine, and serotonin, similar to the effects of antidepressant drugs. The added benefit of regular physical activity is that it is a healthy alternative to these drugs.

Exercise can improve your outlook, your energy levels, and reduce your anxiety and depression. Studies have shown that people who exercise regularly have elevated mood levels and report lower levels of anxiety and depression compared to their inactive counterparts. Not only can you push through that tough workout to keep you accountable to yourself and your goals, but that accountability can carry over to the rest of your day. In other words, getting close and personal with a challenging exercise can make you more likely to stay on task, manage your time better, and less likely to feel swamped by everyday stress.

10.4. Point 4

In essence, emotional stability is the ability to absorb and be resistant to depression, restlessness, and negative emotions. By maintaining physical fitness, one can maintain emotional stability and control mood swings much better. This is because physical fitness is not exclusively about exercise alone; it is also about proper diet, relaxation, and rest. All these would, in turn, have an effect on the levels of serotonin, endorphin, noradrenaline, and dopamine in the bloodstream. Important glands stimulated during exercise are the adrenal glands, the glands responsible for the regulation of serotonin, which in turn causes joy. Such exercises that would stimulate the adrenal glands are lifting weights, yoga, or any type of play.

There is a reason why the philosophers and physicians of old termed human nature as being "holistic". True to this term, health is not only a state of physical wellness; it is also a state of mental wellness. There is a common misconception that being healthy only means maintaining the fitness of one's body. But in reality, people fail to understand that the road to fitness is not complete until that road leads to the health of one's mind and emotions. True happiness and health are a result of emotional, spiritual, physical, and mental wellbeing. Here we look into the 4 such things that must be achieved as a result of one being healthier and fitter.

10.5. Point 5

Get a full body massage. A full body massage has been known to relieve stress and emotional discomfort. Physical pain is often relieved by a good massage. Make it a point to have a minimum of at least a half-hour massage twice a week. People may consider this 'spoiling yourself,' but I consider it taking care of myself. Just as your car needs a tune-up, oil change, and general attention, so must you. There are 206 bones and 800 different muscles in the body, giving the body a full license massage is permission to revitalize its performance. Simply race out using a simple stroke over the muscles. Technique is applied here as it is always optimal to move toward the heart. With all hand grip, you smooth one hand over all the flesh along with bone. Use both hands touching the skin to massage the body. For the back, use the thumb and the rest flat. Try to massage clockwise. Your hands must feel heavy, and they must smooth out the surface using the force of the combined grip of your hands. Take your time. If your arms begin to get tired, use slower strokes.

Perform deep breathing exercises. Focus on your breath and breathe deeply. Continue this for two to five minutes. Deep breathing cleanses your body of toxins. It helps to replenish and clear your mind of misunderstandings. It is a way to relax. When you breathe deeply, you obtain deep sleep. Instead of using drugs such as sleep aids, breathe deeply. Try it. I bet you pass out so fast. To ensure yourself of a deep and peaceful sleep, breathe deeply. You have to use a technique to smell the roses/raw smell; hold it; blow out the candles/fragrance. On each part you are breathing in, breathe in deep so that if you were to smell a rose you'd be sucking all the scent from it to every part of your lung. Hold it so that the lungs are soaking up all that scent. In actuality, your lungs have scent so the hold allows all those scent cells to take up the fragrance. As you blow out, blow out long. The candles or fragrance allows you to breathe out long. Keep doing this, being consistent in duration.

CHAPTER 11

Section 11

A body's beauty or shape is not relative, but rather personal. Crash diets, hours of cardio, and torturing workouts are not a solution to happiness. If your body is the only physical house that you need to live in, why would you want to hurt it? Fitness should not be seen as a punishment for your past or present exercise neglecting, bad eating, and self-despise habits, but rather as a proactive contribution to a better life. By seeing fitness similarly to bathing and eating, you will make time to nourish your body as you should. This will help you to be healthier, to live longer, to cope better with routine obligations, to reduce the chances of suffering from the bad posture caused as a result of years of neglect, and to look better and more vigorous, and consequently, even sexier.

With the arrival of the "selfie generation", it has become increasingly difficult to escape body criticism. Body shaming seems particularly omnipresent on the internet in the form of comments, in everything from content created by everyday people to that developed by professionals. Persons who undergo bullying or body shaming are more likely to develop resentment, hate, and a lack of motivation toward fitness and exercises or any positive change in their life, while those who encourage such hatred may also end up being affected themselves. Studies have shown that those who bully get as much happiness as those who are bullied or shamed under their mean comments.

11.1. Point 1

For a holistic approach to succeed, exercising the mind is as important as exercises to boost fitness. While fitness exercises help us to consciously steer our lives and fitness of consciousness takes us to the fulfillment of this process, mental exercise builds the fitness of the mind, providing inner peace and tranquility. Like the trinity defined, fitness for consciousness, mind, and body is essential for today's busy world. The majority of people live in this world and won't get time to get away. At least they can manage to spare some personal time to address their health issues by practicing multiple styles of exercises. Perhaps, some deeper practices while in the profession could also be carved out. Recommending such practices, YogaSiromani TM Krishnamoorthy of Yoga teacher training in India insisted personal choices appropriately support the right style of practicing these exercises.

Fitness for the mind can be explained with the soap theory. Just as the primary function of soap is to cleanse dirt from the body, fitness of the mind is to cleanse the dirt of worries, concerns, and stress and make the mind stable and calm. The ultimate aim of fitness of the mind is to go beyond all desires and fears, to realize the true nature of oneself. A good body is needed to live and maintain oneself comfortably – without which, one can't proceed on the path of consciousness. Hence, the body has to be kept healthy. But fitness of the body must not be at the expense of overweighing the mind – as the mind is essential to realize the purpose of life. Raman Maharshi in Maharshi's Gospel stressed this point. A healthy and functionally fit body serves as the temple of our essential self or consciousness.

11.2. Point 2

Would you like some suggestions to keep fit? If so, follow the rule of threes, a magical figure. Consider fitting in three 30-minute sessions of muscle training and stretching; walking as your physical activity in three 45-minute sets; and, when it comes to heart disease prevention, three times a week you should keep your target heart rate and respiration rate for at least 20 minutes, remaining at 150 to 190 beats per minute, achieving two units of increased breathing for a cycle without exhaustion. The World Health Organization suggests everyone who can walk all days should move as much as possible, that is, walk, either brisk, slow, or normal, any movement of the body as much as possible, but in a regular part of the daily or weekly routine.

According to the World Health Organization, the following five basic components will help you maintain a healthy life: being healthy improves fitness parameters (strength, endurance, and flexibility), psychological parameters, self-esteem, and health perception. That is, fitness is first and foremost a means for attaining good health. Furthermore, fitness raises mood levels. When you practice, the body secretes endorphins (monamines capable of eliminating pain, reducing bad mood, increasing self-esteem, and providing pleasure). Another important aspect is face-to-face muscle work involving various groups of muscle fibers, increasing one's body contour and improving posture. Aspiration for physical perfection makes you improve your posture and learn how to sit and walk more elegantly. This is how posture improves and, consequently, the breathing becomes more ample and efficient. Improvement, in turn, further raises the fitness conditions, creating a cycle of physical perfection forcing posture and breathing to improve.

11.3. Point 3

Exercise is essential for ensuring that we remain in the best health and that our bodies remain strong enough to keep us safe for as long as possible. Staying healthy also aids with the aging process. As we get older, our bodies become inherently weaker as all natural processes do, but if we spend our younger years effectively looking after our bodies and our minds, it will be a lot easier to deal with the effects of aging when it does become problematic. Incorporate the above-mentioned principles into your life and then see how much healthier and better you feel.

The ancient Greeks had it right with the idea of a sound mind in a sound body. A holistic approach is the best way to ensure a healthy and happy life – treating your body properly through nourishment and exercise is the best critique for treating your mind well through periods of quiet reflection or mindfulness practice. Exercise is essential for ensuring that we remain in the best health and that our bodies remain strong enough to keep us safe for as long as possible. There are many different ways of doing this, you just have to find what works for you. For some, this is gentle exercise such as yoga or swimming, but others are set on adrenaline-fueled hobbies like mountain biking and white-water rafting.

11.4. Point 4

Fitness is known, of course, to depend greatly on genetic makeup. But genetic endowment defines a rough phase space for each person, which the mature and adult form finally inhabits. There are many activities which can be pursued that can help to situate a person in the locale of that phase space where fitness is maximized. First, there are aspects of body function that, with physical activity, are ascertained to perform more effectively. Core strength, flexibility, good aka, and proprioception play an important and positive role in the two environments we must all inhabit: the physical and the mental. Since every thought and interaction is accompanied by the flow of a chemical that floods the body, and exercises with known medical benefits; good cognitive function, memory and restoration, and capacity for analysis and synthesis, and passion, exercises whose benefits in these areas have been documented; emotional stability, exercises whose benefits for this condition are well known. Lastly, associative success which, regardless of its form, will always restore the emotions and general state of well-being.

If a person is living in a way that helps them grow physically, intellectually, and emotionally, then they are leading a life that allows them to enjoy human potential at its best. They must also interact with others who are living in ways that stimulate their energies in a positive way. This presumes that interactions between two persons can affect the fitness of each. If this assumption is correct, then all persons have at least three responsibilities with respect to others: first, do not knowingly harm them (which we have interpreted as meaning that each person's fitness can be affected in a negative way by the actions of another); second, help them as much as possible to be fit; third, always be vigilant of a person's behavioral traits since these help determine their choices and actions no matter how trivial these may seem. Of these three, the second is perhaps the most important, for it simply strengthens the link between the fitness of every person and the environment in which they live. It guarantees that the well-being of a person is dependent not only on their own actions, but also on the actions of everyone else.

11.5. Point 5

There are many different activities that can fall into these three categories. For aerobic activity, think: walking, hiking, bike riding, playing tennis, cardio classes, swimming or jogging. Weightlifting would be the start of resistance training, but it could also include squats, push-ups, lunges, step-ups or anything else that requires force against something else. Flexibility? Yoga, stretching, or tai chi. Honestly, a good physical fitness regimen would include all three of these types of activities. For muscle strength, building better balance, flexibility, and even aerobic benefits, take a yoga class that encourages 3-5 pounds hand weights. While it's not the typically calming yoga experience, it does incorporate the three areas of physical fitness and includes mental imagery as well as breathing techniques.

Turn it into a habit: Participation in physical fitness activity should be made into a habit, so much so that a day should feel odd if it hasn't included some form of exercise. Turn exercise into an appointment. Buy pedometers and walk at least 10,000 steps every day. Assessing your fitness level is a great indicator of the state of your overall health. Participate in a group exercise session or sport of your choice, stay committed to fitness goals, and visualize success. Win in your mind before you win in the gym, and use the power of mental imagery often. The physical effects of training are the result of mental and physical conditioning, so always train hard—never just go through the motions. The mind is a powerful tool in everything you do, so use it to your advantage and strive to do all things to the best of your ability.

CHAPTER 12

Section 12

That's why Boehm thinks it's time to bring fitness back to its true form, the wellness space. That is the place where simple first aid can be made, he expects that this can be a holistic control through the illumination of mental risks and ethical demands that we need. We have in culture today. "Fitness and health is frustrating for most people because it is too serious at first and then it divides too close to the parties," says Boehm. "We would make health to be easier if we aimed for greater health and less fitness. You will feel much less damaging about your health if you make it clearer."Once the soul-on-fire or watchdog attention could be described as a rewarding philosophy or life assuredness. Call it whatever you want, but health professionals and therapists this day know very well that mind and body intertwine all the time and that their influence does in a practical period initiate embryosis conditions. As century came to an end, we knew less and less of the art than the Greeks did. At the same time, we have never received all the benefits of the performance involved.

Fitness expert and wellness coach Wollie Boehm thinks the current fitness culture is improvidence. "It's a shame the way our fitness culture treats our only physical self," he thinks that human are usually adept at studying contrasts: "Expressive buildings, mountains landscaped through the passage of time will even distract us from the perceived mid-engine orange mess visible on a Lamborghini." Yet, with almost being always joined by technology, the three-part speech of mind, body and soul has become at best a two-part discussion.

12.1. Point 1

There's nothing like physical exertion to wake up our minds and alter our attitudes. Studies have shown that physical exercise is directly related to improved brain health. Individuals who are physically active have been shown to have improved brain functions. Overall, mental functions such as thinking, learning, and judgment are improved and maintained in those who utilize exercise instead of those who live a sedentary lifestyle. Endorphins, neurotransmitters in the brain responsible for a good mood and natural pain relief, are stimulated during exercise, enhancing mental health. It doesn't take running a marathon to become endowed with a better attitude. More modest forms of physical activity may only need to be completed regularly to show their investment in your overall health. Aerobic exercises which only require moderate intensity, like walking, for a mere thirty minutes can improve mood and reduce symptoms commensurate to anxiety and depression. Yoga improves mental health, not just supplying physical benefits. Mindful movement and attention to the breath enhance mental conditions. Participants in a study showed improvement in anxiety, depression, hostilities, and concerns after practicing yoga many times a week for a couple of months. Additionally, dedicating 15 minutes of your day to go for a walk while interacting with nature significantly decreased negative intrusions.

It's not breaking news that mental health and physical health are deeply intertwined. Living a lifestyle conducive to optimal health can lead to greater physical health which, in turn, helps individuals address and even prevent mental health issues. In this article, I'll be going into how living healthfully can bring out the best in ourselves and enhance our lives in four different categories: physical, nutritional, mental, and social health. The time to begin implementing healthy habits is now. It isn't easy, and no one is perfect all the time, but life is a marathon, not a sprint, and even the smallest steps yield benefits.

12.2. Point 2

In this sense of community, don't be afraid to ask for help or share advice with someone else. Not only does it help to foster a positive atmosphere, but it also can help to introduce you to some like-minded people in your gym or community. Learning from others and offering help are great ways to expand your fitness perspective and opens countless doors for you to achieve success. Once you have been working out for a while and you feel strong and positive, don't ever forget how you felt on that very first day you returned to your new lifestyle – insecurities and uncertainties are still a part of the daily struggle for some who look up to you. Not only will your arrival illustrate that the pursuit of health and fitness is not a fool's dream, but it will also illustrate that it is driven by all sorts of different people with different experiences and motivators.

To stay motivated and to see results, being in a fun and engaging environment while working out is important. Working out in a positive environment is not only motivating, but it is also healthy. Happy people are less likely to fall ill, and the less ill a person is, the better result is expected from a person's workout. When people are in a good mood, they are more likely to work harder, making a workout even more effective in achieving personal goals. It is undeniable that success is a matter of mindset – a mindset that helps carry you through the stress of a workday, through the wilting mid-day slump or the almost overwhelming 2:30 feeling. Once you eliminate the self-pity that gets most people down, you will not only feel more empowered to power through a difficult day, but you will also feel like you can take on the world. This is an immeasurably invaluable part of the gym experience.

12.3. Point 3

There are concrete steps you can take to help you think through and identify what your reason is for committing to a healthier lifestyle and why your experience will be different from the myriad of people who've failed in the past. One of the best ways to define a clear and specific reason is by first realizing what you don't want in life anymore. Once you've hit rock bottom, then it's an ideal condition because that very conviction will drive you to act in an irreversible direction.

Sinek writes, "The WHY is the purpose, cause, or belief that drives every one of us." He goes on to emphasize the fact that we're all drawn to individuals and companies who are purposeful, having a strong reason – and not just a reactive cause. "That conviction is the best way to differentiate an individual or an organization, and the strength of that conviction will be the difference that decides whether or not it's sustainable."

It was Simon Sinek who introduced me to the concept of knowing your why and having a good reason for doing what you choose to do every day. As he elaborates at length in his book, he suggests that everyone who has any idea about what success is and how to achieve it always starts with the essential question – WHY? This singular focus for your reason for waking up every day ultimately forces you to develop a very specific plan for how you spend your hours.

12.4. Point 4

This book is meant to guide you on your journey to holistic wellness, which, to me, means that how you treat your mind and your body acts sort of like a circle. When you make the optimal decision for your physical health, you are making the optimal decision for your mental health and vice versa. When you are kind and understanding with your thoughts, you are more likely to make the optimal decision when you are at risk. If you take a few extra minutes a day to do something you love, that adds up to something you love doing. There is an intricate connection between how you treat your mind and how you treat your body; this relationship is different for everyone, and it expands throughout each of the twelve points made throughout the duration of this book.

You were not breathed into life just to pay bills and die. I firmly believe that you were put on this earth to find purpose in everything you do, accomplish dreams, and form a strong connection with other people. Whether you think that your purpose is to create a product that revolutionizes the industry, to travel, to teach, to be the father of two, or to spread a message, there is a reason for every action you decide to take. On that note, there is a reason why you're reading this right now.

12.5. Point 5

We all agree that "Knowledge is Power". Since then, many ideas have been transformed into knowledge. This is especially true of psychological and physical fitness. In this article, we shall provide norms for healthy living and improvements, as also work to improve knowledge. Knowledge is made more accessible and useful to you and your family. It is designed for a family, not experts or enthusiasts. Therefore, we have deliberately avoided expert jargon and removed many steps typically undertaken by trained professionals. While developing this plan, for simplicity, even the scientific evidence has been considerably reduced. However, everything presented is based on more than one published scientific paper. We then applied that knowledge to improve body composition and health. More generally, the same principles were applied to psychological health, eventually to develop a generalized strategy. We finally derived a simple calculator-based strategy that you can use. A "first step" of a family into a long-term better future.

We believe that the path to total fitness is through better knowledge. We will teach you how to improve your mind and body. You will also receive concrete tools for learning and training both. PHR will continue to guide you on your path of self-improvement. An incremental improvement strategy is presented. Total fitness can be achieved through better knowledge. A generalized plan of this strategy is presented based on known scientific publications. You can calculate your current BMI and predicted body weight. A science-based strategic plan, if followed, will result in your desired body weight and improved health. Knowledge is made more accessible and useful to you and your family.

CHAPTER 13

Section 13

First, focus on music in your life. Music has an amazing effect on our brain. We all enjoy a type of music in our own way, and it turns out that the music we like opens more complex and connected networks in our brain. Essentially, the music is helping our brain to think in ways that are more advanced than what we can normally think of. This, in turn, helps develop more analytical thinking, which directly relates to our problem-solving skills. This adds a great connection between what we can relate to in life and how we solve those problems. Music makes a lot of sense to interactively help us understand life in a variety of ways. This, in turn, develops better overall health for the way we solve life's circumstances.

You need to have some form of exercise program and eat right for better health. However, you can have all that and still feel "empty" inside. Let's look at some ways to address this nagging issue and help you achieve a better sense of overall completeness. I will be the first to admit that you do have to have some form of exercise program in your life to help your brain function well, and eating healthy does contribute to your overall well-being. However, let's look at some additional methods that you can use to be a better you. Here are twelve ideas for your mind and body health. These tips are intended to be a set of collective ideas for your all-around health.

13.1. Point 1

Point 2: Filter. Keep what you fancy. As I mentioned above, trying to fit into diet plans can be a nightmare. Each diet plan comes with fancy words like 'Fat-burning-foods' and 'Muscle-building-Foods' or the more common references - 'Calories', 'Carbs', 'Fats', 'Proteins'. The main things you want to do is cutting processed sugars and ridiculous amounts of unhealthy fats from your diet and consume the right amount of proteins to convert fat into muscle. And of course, don't starve yourself either. Why does this seem like a secret recipe to some people? I know, it seems simple for a majority of you out there. If you are one of us who break into a cold sweat upon hearing these words, I understand. That's how difficult these notions are being marketed. Remember, the best nutrition comes from balanced meals. You don't need to force yourself to eat something that makes you gag because the internet told you it's good for you (And, assuming you did eat it, chances are, you'll be miserable after having a meal you don't like).

Point 1: Keep it simple. We might have an idea of a healthy diet in our minds - low in sugars, rich in proteins, moderate amounts of complex carbs and unsaturated fats. But we end up complicating it. There are innumerable diet plans that tell you to prepare elaborate meals with expensive and hard to find ingredients. God save you if you have allergies or intolerances to a couple of things. You are heading straight into a nightmare when you are sticking to cooking instructions from different meal plans. Start off simple - wholesome food, hygienically prepared, consumed in timely intervals. As you discover more about what's needed for your body and your skills improve, you could graduate to preparing meals with more complex ingredients.

13.2. Point 2

Over time, the brain's susceptibility to issues of mental-physical health has been recognized. From the morphological point of view (on the existence of angiogenesis, i.e. zonal fixation areas of the hippocampus in aerobic sports) or from the functional point of view (an increased number of dopaminergic receptors, which is a measure of cerebral plasticity in the event of doing a sport; concerning genetics, for example, physical exercise modulates neural mechanisms - the BDNF gene contributes to synaptic plasticity and membrane stability). In this sense, whatever the neural level, the motor component is strongly solicited when mental functions are confronted with the challenge of change. This is why from a practical point of view, the famous phrase of Jean Paccini "we can only understand what we have built" is very well adapted to what numerous researchers show about the conditions of the acquisition of new knowledge. The difficulty of acquiring knowledge lies above all in the monotony that can be perceived by subjects who sometimes have behaviors close to "lab rats" when they feel nothing more than a number for the experimenter and no longer an individual with a specific potentiality.

The expression "mens sana in corpore sano" (a sound mind in a sound body) by the Roman poet Juvenal is quite relevant in our discussion. Your mind is also a vital part of your fitness and wellness, so both must be in harmony. This harmonious state, based on the benefits of regular physical exercise, practicing meditation, and a good diet, can be called mental-physical or holistic wellness. Indeed, many benefits can be achieved if we pay attention to our mental-physical health. However, this problem is generally viewed as someone's personal concern. What about companies where many people spend their lives? They should also pay attention to their employees' mental-physical health. In this study, we aim to support this vision, first by emphasizing the benefits of physical activity. We do not claim here that sport is good for you, but rather that, other things being equal, if you practice a sport regularly, you will "suffer" less and feel better.

13.3. Point 3

It's of course a deliberate distraction, something to easily consume and a great market for charlatans; including the no talent lucky people we call celebrities, who by looking good dictate standards and dumb us down, the essence of real living quoting words and 2nd hand wisdom from philosophers, politicians, scientists and abstracted poetry they never even heard of. Lest we remember, Leonardo Da Vinci, Mother Teresa, Einstein, Isaac Newton, Steve Jobs, Archimedes and many others weren't the icon of physical attractiveness in deceitful comparison to the likes of present unimportant characters for they were masters of the mind, they were self educated and self explored individuals, open minded, creative, self disciplined, ambitious and continually pursuing and reaching success, helping and contributing to society.

Have you noticed that there isn't a correlation between beautiful facial features or the ideal body type and lasting marriages or relationships? We all have friends who are in happy stable relationships, yet according to social norms shouldn't be; norm dictates that perfect facial features and a catwalk body are the main characteristics one should/have to look for in a potential partner and if that's lacking and god forbid so is age, a relationship of this kind is usually seen as "just a fling, the fun's over, short lived and not a wise grab". Research after research and testimony after testimony show without a doubt that there is no real correlation. The physical is superficial and doesn't only fade with time but most times is deceiving for real potential circumstances. Yet we continue only focusing on this aspect of our being as if it were the most important facet of the human nature.

13.4. Point 4

How important is physical health? It is extremely important, in fact absolutely paramount. If your health deteriorates, your plans, dreams, aspirations, and major portions of your everyday lives will come to a rough halt. We all want to travel the journey of life with joy, purpose, and with each day taking us closer to the goal. Such a journey is possible only when you are in the best of health. The necessity of physical fitness is based on two vital facts – that in virtually every work, a substantial level of fitness to some extent is necessary and that without it, the mind and body can't function optimally. When do we feel the keenest desire to live? When we are in the prime of our health. The greatest joy in life comes from good health. When the morning sun paints nature with its resplendent beauty, the accomplishment of any dreams or aspirations we have depends entirely on the strength, energy, and vivacity we gain from good health.

"The greatest wealth is health," wrote Seneca, yet most of us tend to take this most crucial aspect of our lives for granted. We are all familiar with the numerous health benefits of regular physical activity. Regular exercise reduces the risk of often life-threatening diseases. It promotes healthy body weight, improves immune function and keeps our hearts healthy, reduces the risk of cancer and diabetes, lowers cortisol levels, and offers many mental health benefits, such as reducing anxiety and depression, increasing our sense of well-being and bolstering our perception of cognitive functions. None of us can afford to ignore these benefits; they are essential building blocks in each of our lives.

13.5. Point 5

Some researchers believe that the life and functional potency of new life are influenced by the maternal effects of the quality of life that the maternal environment provides to the baby in her uterus.

With the realization that a unified biology of the processes that create and consume energy can impact the offspring, the importance of communication between the processes or aspects of lifestyle factors could eventually improve the regulation of the availability of nutrients and hormonal signals to the fetus in both safe and non-devastating times for the mother and/or fetus. This perspective is unique in the intention of delaying the onset of chronic diseases in newborns by correcting aspects of our lifestyle (the development of disease processes, up to $\geq$ 18/20 years) that we have contributed to the environment (the mother's and her offspring's metabolic health over a period of 9 months) in which the sperm and egg are fertilized.

The term "fitness" refers to one's physical and mental well-being. It is no longer news that unfit individuals are prone to recurrent diseases, and that children born to unhealthy parents (whether due to inactivity or other physical or mental problems) are born with known (e.g., heart disease or diabetes) or idiopathic diseases (for which they have an unknown genetic predisposition or developmental risk factors, not due to infection or vaccines). There is increasing evidence that the body needs complex physical and mental stimuli from the prenatal period to prevent conditions that lead to morbidity and poor health in young age, old age, and senile age. Today's society needs more people who make use of their functional potential and stay fit, as there is no age when exercising (physical and cognitive fitness) is contraindicated.

CHAPTER 14

Section 14

Completely acknowledge and accept the truth that 06.13am is forever lost, but everything from 06am is forever kept. Reason: 6 stands for Anja Chakra (purity, initiative, wisdom) and 13(Higher plane of existence) – out of mind but wisdom is forever retained. Since mind clogs piling up in the past need depth of wisdom for purification. So randomly during the day, few seconds make the effort to take five conscious breaths, silently chant shubh (auspicious). This applies equally to stress givers and stress takers but unsought interruptions should not be encouraged. Anu – is anu individual, not sub-atomic/mind atom. The five conscious breaths purify mind, removing the subtle mind particles.

These few dis-jointed thoughts are the essence of Yoga Sutra 4:34. If anyone finds the conceptual framework worth a try, please acknowledge understanding since there is no bar to 'copy right'. E.D. Wow! Yes! But do ensure confidentiality and first personally apply it. This 'unique' package (enable Yoga Sutra Asanas, celebrate life, fitness is freedom, and regulate body temperature, budhi, intelligence) should not tempt anyone. It is primarily a loner's world for self-introspection, and take off an hour, for a half hour, as a try, at least for one day a week or every morning/evening. Remember – versatility, focus, spontaneity, specificity, it is all anaerobic – when bent the stretch is better felt.

14.1. Point 1

Acquiring knowledge and new skills is a part of self-improvement. Whether it is mastering your science project, giving a good presentation, or learning a new sales technique at work, learning improves your understanding of the world and can help you accomplish more. Maintaining the philosophy of using mind and body as the basis for my fitness methods, a holistic approach must not stop. Continue growing, communicating, and connecting with others, just as one important physical fitness aspect connects to another. I am forever devoted to ongoing fitness and self-improvement by teaching and trying various solutions and expanding my mastery of my profession of personal training and group fitness.

The above refers to the belief that exercise should go further than just getting your body in shape, but actually developing your mind and fostering self-improvement. Exercise and physical fitness are not isolated events, and the mind-body connection and its benefits are provable, powerful factors in training and health. The majority may not completely appreciate the ripple effect of how sitting for long periods influences physical fitness in a negative way.

Everyone uses personal time to do what is important for enhancing personal happiness, part of which is long-term health and applicable physical fitness. In preserving this harmony, I train my clients and create the direction for their day-to-day fitness. The importance of using the intellect in fixing the body has the power to increase the effectiveness of exercise and the body's ability to maintain key fitness. This article displays just a taste of what is applicable to overall health within my training and information guiding. It will be very challenging to include all of my related philosophy to fitness. A person will have to communicate with me directly to witness much of that.

14.2. Point 2

Mental and physical fitness are not just two linked concepts; they are tied in a knot called you. You eat for both the body and the mind; you cook and taste with your physical and mental dexterity. Physical well-being is a precursor to mental peace. In addition, the quality of your mental health depends on the physical health. Mental and physical health are linked and this has been observed for centuries. War and famine have their particular toll on the health of the people. In times of war, the number of psychiatric patients can multiply manifold. The sufferers of mental diseases find it almost impossible to go on normal life activities, e.g. go for shopping, eat healthy food, and take regular exercise.

Mental health can be compromised by the existence of other diseases, such as hepatitis. The common causative lifestyle factors of the non-communicable diseases are also responsible for poor mental health. The biological factors, which are a cause of coronary artery disease and colon cancer, are the identical causes of the symptoms of poor mental health and a low state of psychological well-being. By adjusting our lifestyle, we can reduce the risk of both non-communicable diseases and poor mental health. Therefore, the focus on the promotion of mental health should be much broader and should also incorporate the promotion of lifestyle-related factors both related to physical and psychological health.

14.3. Point 3

Yoga is a social, spiritual, and physical practice that aims to transform the body and mind. The ultimate aim of yoga is to reach the state of self-awareness, inner peace, and spiritual recognition. This is achieved by training the body and the mind through a wisdom method. Literally, the term yoga came from a Sanskrit root that conveys the notion of union. Yoga is the process to synergize perfectly the physical, vital, mental, emotional, psychic, and intellectual human facet with the soul or the real self.

Yoga, in a more down-to-earth perspective, is an integrated approach having physical movements and postures (asanas - physical dimension), breathing exercises (pranayama - vital dimension), intellectual and emotional management and control (mental and emotional bodies), meditation, chanting, devotion, rituals, etc. (psychic or subliminal and spiritual dimensions) to maintain and restore the health and harmony of a person and for self-awareness.

A session of yoga usually starts with the practitioner first concentrating, warming up or limbering, and subsequently rehearsing a meticulously designed and effervescently prescribed set of postures - asanas (physical dimension) combined with breathing exercises (pranayama) in getting into a state of tranquility, thereby facilitating meditative or psychic or spiritual practices, followed by relaxation. An important feature of the practice methodology of yoga is that, under the guidance of a competent guru or a teacher, one learns how to perform each asana precisely, the order in which to perform them, and how to coordinate the breathing pattern with the practice, ensuring the full effect of yoga practices on the body, breath, and mind.

While the ancient practices of yoga were associated with spirituality (transcendence from false knowledge, bondage, and entanglements to a life of happiness, freedom, and liberation), regular practices of yoga aid a person in maintaining a state of equanimity and being refreshed and rejuvenated at the physical and mental levels. Physical yoga is an essential component of holistic living, ensuring physical fitness, mental agility, and emotional stability.

14.4. Point 4

A panic attack occurs as a result of the body's fight-or-flight (or somewhere in between) mechanism. It is a result of being caught in the loop of anxiety, which results in the production of excessive cortisol. The sequence of chemical reactions triggered off as a result can finally be debilitating to the body and manifest as symptoms such as breathlessness, chest pain, palpitations, dizziness, and temperature changes. These symptoms themselves can infuse more terror into the patient's mind and make him visualize the worst (fatal heart attack). Thus, a stream of catastrophic thoughts keeps the panic attack alive even beyond the expectation of the body's fight-or-flight mechanism.

Some of the routes by which the body can learn to desensitize itself from this repeated exposure to panic and anxiety are: 1) Maintain a healthy diet: Remember that undigested food particles are the primary source of inflammatory mediators that finally reach the brain, thereby potentially increasing anxiety. 2) Have frequent but small meals: This avoids stress on the gastrointestinal tube and also avoids hypoglycemia and dehydration, which can potentiate anxiety in a patient who is already prone. 3) Avoid caffeine: It is not the greatest idea to bombard the already anxious brain with a surge of adrenaline and cortisol via caffeine. 4) Take some foods rich in omega 3 fatty acids: Omega 3 fatty acids can provide resiliency to the still forming brain by fortifying the lipid bilayer membranes in the outermost extensions of the neuron known as the axons. The resulting sturdiness of the neuron aids in electrical signal propagation and will confer resistance to further anxiety. 5) Maintain a routine of regular exercise: A routine of regular exercise can promote the growth of neurons in the hippocampus, which is the primary center of emotion regulation in the brain. This would only mean much greater resiliency to the stresses that the body will be subject to. During exercise, the brain, via the production of endorphins, can also induce a calming effect, and thus several exercise routines are increasingly being incorporated in psychotherapeutic regimens for treating anxiety.

14.5. Point 5

Acupuncture, Ayurveda, magnet therapy, homeopathy, and energy healing (Reiki) are all complex, holistic interventions that are recognized for their role in healing the mind, body, and spirit. Often these traditional arts are placed in the category of 'alternative methods' with the assumption that many are 'unscientific'. However, research is slowly providing evidence for their efficacy as integrative sciences. A comprehensive study of scientific evidence concludes, "all 5 CAM therapies have reported high levels of patient satisfaction. Their potential for clinical efficacy remains relatively high, and meta-analyses, when available, do often report positive results". The use of 'alternative' therapies is no longer as rare as it was ten years ago. The continued use of these therapies in rapidly expanding numbers across the world is due to their effectiveness, replicating the words of a distinguished physicist and polymath, John Coan, that "we have to accept what 'works' whether our current scientific theories can account for it or not". The benefits of these methods need to be critically appraised and harnessed for the betterment of society, not with skepticism and questions about its mechanism of action but by harnessing the goodness and holistic approach it brings, completing the present scientific theory and methodology. It is time to integrate modern scientific methods with traditional knowledge, bringing the two together through consistent interfacing and research.

Research has suggested that these CAMs (Complementary and Alternative Medicines) seem to exhibit their healing effects through multiple pathways on the organ systems of the body. Interactions between the mind, body, brain, and social adaptation systems are ever so profound. Thus, it is important for individuals to bring about a strong relationship between these elements of the body, as a place for the manifestation of their higher self. Consequently, holistic therapies that help the individual work in agreement with these naturally existing systems bring about the popular notion of 'finding the right balance'. Due to the strong interwoven network of tissues and organs, it comes as no surprise that therapies aimed at the mind, brain, and interaction strength between mind and body can modulate functions in these organ systems. Thus, a therapeutic process that engages several components of the body could lead to a more profound healing.

CHAPTER 15

Section 15

Simple as it may be, to prioritize activities of the fitness concept, significantly intervening to evolve and mainly in promoting continuous physical training in order to identify the need to lay most effort improving the physical health and body image of the future, in an incorporeal and indirect way there are benefits of time, protection, income gain, training assembly and/or products, emotional and psychological practices, in addition to spiritual and cultural aspects that also act directly and indirectly in improving the proper functioning of the body structure. Attending directly, in constructively adjusting programs in an ample field called complementary activities to the fitness concept, may use techniques, interventions, means, instruments, thoughts, knowledge, investigation and disciplined and religious organization beyond perception to increase the quality of health of the traditionally considerate parameters.

Going to the gym, getting in shape, and paying particular attention in general to one's physical health may often be motivated by many factors. Some of these factors may be to feel confident in appearance because of selective body enhancement, to keep up with an attractive lifestyle that is lived by some member of family, friend, society or Hollywood celebrity, or to prevent illness, and in that way avoid complications that may deteriorate physical and health quality of life. That is why the accomplishment of an excellent physical health is done almost exclusively through training of the most evident physical characteristics directly affected by the easiest measurable metabolic and functional exercise parameters naturally observable: physical endurance (aerobic) and muscle strength and endurance (anaerobic). Technically within the essence of these three types there are many exercises, various routine methods, and types of movement to attend to the large variety of the human body anatomical form and capacities of structure (metabolism), allied with space for many activities and contributions directed by scientists, professionals, organized practices, material, and procedures focused on the many genres in all age groups.

15.1. Point 1

That said, we still have people who, despite feeling the need and being convinced of the benefits, find an excuse to just sit back and do nothing about it (rather than returning to feeling sorry for themselves). For most of us, this involves some or more of the following: lack of willpower, poor time management, lack of motivation, and absence of self-discipline. It is hard, no one says otherwise. Despite the number of phenomenal benefits that exercise guarantees, the number of people who engage in it continues to diminish over time. Even regular people who love to exercise need help to stay motivated. You do not have to do it all in one go; if it becomes boring, do what you enjoy most first. Alternatively, you could consider engaging a yoga instructor, personal trainer, or participating in advantageous activities like team sports. You could sign up at a gym or buy a membership subscription for a specialized fitness program to start shedding off fat or further develop as a bodybuilder.

Exercise in any form has the power to alleviate depression, anxiety, and other thoughts that create a heavy mind. This happens as a result of different chemical (hormonal and neurotransmitter) levels reaching their ideal equilibrium briefly during and for long after physical exercise. The type, duration, intensity, and frequency of exercise usually determine the level of chemical balance and the amount of energy expended. A secondary benefit of exercise is a transformation that begins to take place in the body. The individual may not necessarily experience a loss in body fat or muscle gain, but they may experience an increased ability to perform more dynamic aspects of everyday tasks, a reduced risk of disease, a better and longer night's sleep, and so on.

15.2. Point 2

When someone engages in a regular physical fitness program, a transformed body will emerge because with improved physical health, the loops between the two essential elements of their being (mind and body) become balanced. The body through the mind is better able to serve its owner. When the body is able to serve its owner, the mind will continue to direct this energy, taking odd parts shaped or easily molded by the hands of someone who needs new resolve. If we allow our physical shape to remain unruly and unadaptive - we are unwise in engaging in activities relative to other external affairs. However, we should not underestimate the relationships between these two essential elements. It is important that we remember, frequent exercise and proper physical nourishment and care trump sedentary behavior, unhealthy food consumption, and a lack of sleep. Refraining from this unhealthy lifestyle is essential as it promotes growth, development, and contrasts a negative pattern of continued degeneration.

Mental wellness requires physical wellness, and vice versa. Our mind and body are connected. When we improve our physical health, our mental health improves as well. Regular exercise can boost our self-esteem, help us to set goals and achieve them, take our minds off of worries, and improve our sleep. With increased physical activity, our bodies experience reduced muscle tension, stimulation of the production of endorphins (the body's natural painkiller), enhancement of our mood, and a boost in our self-image. Regular physical activity will often lead to an improved fitness level, which will also positively impact the health of our brain. Experts in Brainhealth at the University of Illinois state that exercise is associated with changes in certain chemicals in the brain. The chemicals associated with the stress response are reduced by regular physical activity. Exercise also leads to changes in the brain's architecture, and that can affect mood and essentially promote a more calming, stress-free existence. Exercise basically helps the brain to block out distracting stressful information, allowing our mind to focus on the tasks at hand.

15.3. Point 3

Yet, the terms 'holistic', 'holism' or 'whole person' are rarely included in the titles of wellness programs that include both the psychological and the kinesiological aspects of health, despite the growing consensus on the importance of such a holistic approach to mental and physical health; rather, such holistic programs often are included in repression or self-regulation therapy or in health and fitness programs that attempt to change the lifestyles of individuals with mental health problems, such as Wellness Recovery Action Plan (WRAP) or in the rapidly growing field of 'mental health promotion'. Such programs often do not address all aspects of mental health, however, and performance of psychomotor exercises is often not the main part of these programs.

What is a holistic approach to better mental and physical health? A wellness program designed to improve physical health often focuses on the improvement of specific components of health, such as the cardiovascular system, the muscles, the joints, or the ability to perform specific motor skills. Similarly, a program designed to improve mental health also generally focuses on specific aspects of mental health, such as the advancement of specific cognitive skills, proclaiming 'mental' health to embody cognitive health alone. However, the idea of holistic health (the belief that overall life balance, including physical, mental, social, and sometimes also spiritual aspects, is essential for personal well-being and that the indicators of a well state are the individual functioning and the wellness of the individual as a whole) is not new to modern psychology. The Greek physician and philosopher Hippocrates (c. 460 - c. 370 BC), for example, states in his work Law ("Prorrhetics"), 27 'For a man, one should always consult a complete vision of his individual as a whole'.

15.4. Point 4

It is important to note that the two aspects are inseparable - one cannot solely focus on the physical and pay no attention to the mental - or vice versa - focusing solely on mental health and ignoring the physical. Author Reiss (2005) in a research paper titled: 'How to Build Employee Morale and Motivation on a Shoestring Budget' - discusses employee motivation and morale. Both important elements to employee happiness and by extension the happiness of the employer. Morale and motivation must come from within. Employers must work on their relationships with their employees. Fitness in both areas is what the employer may modestly expect from the employees. The importance of the mind is further underpinned by CIPD (2009) in its research report titled: Leadership-employee relationships, employee intercultural effectiveness and stress management in UK organizations. Recent years have seen an increasing trend towards holistic wellbeing programmes.

There is a growing concern regarding the mental and physical wellbeing of employees in the workplace - of which the effects on the business at large are undeniable. Employers are taking heed of this growing concern and have implemented a number of far-sighted 'wellbeing' programmes. Most of these programmes focus either on the physical or the mental aspect, however, for true benefit to be achieved, it is suggested that these wellbeing programmes should rather be holistic in nature - that is, they should focus on wellness of both mind and body, with the knowledge that the two are inseparable. This paper takes a holistic approach to employee wellbeing and reviews available research on the subject - with practical methods on how to implement the holistic approach in the work space. The importance of work-life balance is discussed as a prerequisite to the holistic approach.

15.5. Point 5

The work of cognitive functions is based on associative and synaptic relations of neurons. Without the motor functions of the skeletal muscle apparatus, rich accurate and fine regulation, moved by the cortex, these connections do not develop and strengthen. With the active motor areas performance, development is observed in the front part of the brain, which is responsible for understanding and the implementation of models in motion. Therefore, for cognitive development, specialist, speech therapist, and psychologist Pestalozzi proposed a Games and Physical Development System method, which is the development of universities and schools. Movement is an essential condition for efficient (desirable) knowledge, abilities, and skills to be formed. The whole body participates in speech development, the voice is the combined work of essentially all organs, and movement is an expression and basis of development. Therefore, this sees speech, which is the basis of thought, as well as the basis of logic.

There are numerous scientific views on the synthesis of the arts and sports, psychotherapy, dance, singing, exercise therapy, and various techniques to calm and restore the nervous system. For example, a psychologist and specialist in exercise therapy, P. Fratkin, made a concise statement: "For each patient, a diet must be balanced, that is, dancing and singing are necessary." Beautifully put and true! After all, if for some reason a person cannot perform complex movements, which include art (even simple motion includes an element of plastic art - drawing, music - rhythm, and poetry - rhymed speech), it is necessary to give them dancing music. In principle, there are a great deal of techniques of "physical relaxation" - even simple shaking and waving works very well.

For centuries, it was said that "Mens Sana in Corpore Sano" - a healthy mind in a healthy body. This is not just a statement, but a rule to live by. Health is not only the absence of illness, but a state of complete balance of mind and body. For full fitness, it is not enough just to train the physical body, but also the mind. Such a comprehensive approach allows us to achieve the best result and get joy from the process.

Conclusion

In conclusion, the research confirms and supports my hypothesis that mental fitness and body fitness naturally enhance the human potential for obtaining and maintaining improved mental, physical, and emotional health that resonates throughout the body as a holistic approach to a better you. The dual creation and growth of mental fitness and body fitness through consciousness and the synchronization of the correct principles of fitness training articulate the necessity of a holistic approach in creating a better and improved you. This chapter constitutes the fact that different paths in life lead to different claims or goals and in order to achieve those claims or goals, physical and spiritual fitness are equally important in attaining and maintaining one's mental, physical, and emotional intelligence of improved health that resonates throughout the entire body through a holistic approach to a better and improved you. Therefore, as evolution teaches, a holistic approach to mental training for the body and physical training for the spirit rooted in consciousness is needed for successfully achieving healthier mental, physical, and emotional intelligence in an organic and coherent way that resonates throughout the entire human being for improved health and also the human potential.